Contents

What is asthma?

Most people would recognise asthma in a child or adult as attacks of wheezy breathlessness, sometimes on exertion, sometimes at rest, sometimes mild, sometimes severe. Some would recognise specific 'triggers' – for example, animals, fumes, pollens. Some might think of asthma as a condition of children, some as a condition able to affect someone of any age. Some would regard it as an occasional nuisance requiring intermittent treatment only, others as a persistent, significant problem needing continuous treatment. Surely they can't all be right?

In a way they can, although it is this wide range of factors involved in asthma that makes it difficult to come up with a simple definition.

The word 'asthma' is used as a blanket term to cover a condition characterised by episodes of breathlessness caused by intermittent narrowing of the bronchial tubes – or

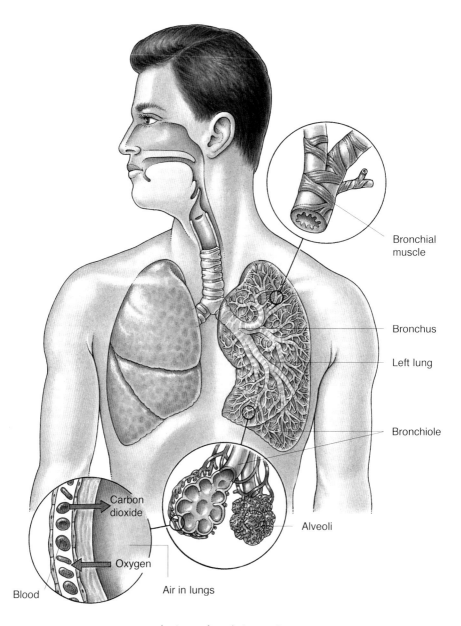

Bronchial muscle

Bronchus

Left lung

Bronchiole

Carbon dioxide

Oxygen

Alveoli

Blood

Air in lungs

Anatomy of respiratory system.
(The main windpipe, bronchi and bronchioles are known as 'the airways'.)

narrow, reducing airflow through them and making the individual breathless and/or wheezy.

This sensitivity of the airways enjoys the medical label 'bronchial hyper-reactivity'. In the surgery or clinic doctors use the term 'twitchy tubes'!

So asthma is not one disease: it covers a multitude of different patterns. Like the word 'cancer' it tells you roughly what sort of condition we are dealing with, what ballpark we are in. Under that general heading you will find a range of severities, a range of triggering factors and a range of outcomes. It logically follows that what is good for one asthmatic person may be unsuitable for another.

airways – within the lung. There are many factors that contribute to the development of asthma in the first instance and many that can induce attacks. In addition, these will vary from individual to individual.

The best definition is that asthma is a condition in which the airways within the lung are inflamed and so are more sensitive to specific factors (triggers) that cause the airways to

Asthma is a very individual condition and management needs to be personalised because of the variety of factors that underlie each individual's asthma.

KEY POINTS

✓ Asthma is not one disease. Like the word 'cancer' it covers a multitude of different patterns

✓ Because of the wide range of factors involved in causing asthma and the variety of responses the body's airways make, it is not easy to define asthma simply

How much asthma is there?

The short answer is – a lot! Up-to-date estimates suggest that 15 per cent of children of primary school age and around 6–7 per cent of the general population in the UK suffer from asthma. It is the commonest condition to be found in Western populations, affecting over three million individuals in England and Wales alone. In children, boys are twice as frequently affected as girls, while in adult life the condition is slightly more common in women.

Is asthma increasing?

Asthma has increased over the past two decades, regardless of what measure of asthma you look at. For example, between the mid-1970s and the early 1990s, there was around a five-fold increase in the numbers of patients presenting to their GP with an attack of asthma, particularly in children. There was also an increase in hospital admissions up to the early 1990s, again particularly in children, possibly reflecting the fact that parents are more likely to seek medical advice for their children than for themselves, although other factors are also likely to play a part. Gratifyingly, the rise has seemed to flatten out since the early 1990s.

Reasons for the increase

It is possible that some of the increase is due to doctors now using the word 'asthma' whereas before they would have used 'wheezy bronchitis', but this cannot explain the greater part of the rise. Exposure to allergens in the home, viral infections, aspects of the indoor environment such as central heating, air pollution, the stress of modern living – even the treatment used for asthma itself – have all been blamed for the increase. However, evidence for any of these individually being responsible is limited. In fact, it is highly likely that the rise is due to a combination of these factors and, in the end, may be quite difficult to sort out.

Deaths

Fortunately, death from asthma is not common. In the mid-1960s a short-lived epidemic of deaths caused by asthma occurred which some thought might be the result of a toxic effect of one of the asthma inhalers on sale at the time. This has been disputed over the years and other factors may have been of importance; it is unlikely that we shall ever know the complete story surrounding that event.

In fact, most asthma deaths are caused by undertreatment of patients and it has been shown that two-thirds of asthma deaths would have been preventable with adequate treatment.

Lately, there has been a further slight rise in asthma deaths in patients over the age of 50 although this, again, settled down in the 1990s. Why this has occurred is not clear, although in the older patient differentiating between asthma and chronic bronchitis is often difficult and this may have led to a change in diagnostic fashion.

Geographical differences in asthma

There are certainly some parts of the UK where asthma admissions and GP attendances are more common and

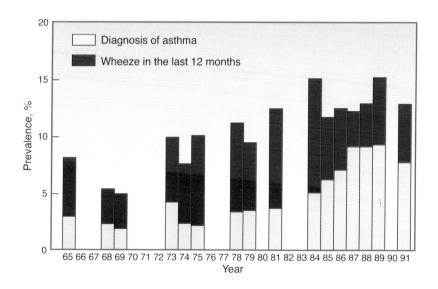

The prevalence of asthma (the proportion of the population who have the condition at any given point in time) has increased since the 1970s – at least among children. (Courtesy of the Lung & Asthma Information Agency.)

other areas where they are less so. However, the differences are modest and do not form a clear-cut geographical pattern, unlike attacks of acute bronchitis, which are higher in the north, becoming less so towards the south. Although the differences within the UK are slight, there are quite huge differences in the distribution of asthma in different parts of the world. It is almost unheard of in Eskimos and black Africans living in rural areas, whereas in the Western Caroline Islands nearly 50 per cent of the inhabitants have asthma, with three-quarters of children being affected.

Between these extremes are the westernised populations such as people in the UK, Australia, New Zealand and other European countries, which all have roughly the same amount of asthma. Interestingly, those parts of the world with less asthma are those that are less encouraging to the survival of the house dust mite.

KEY POINTS

✓ Over three million individuals in England and Wales alone have asthma

✓ Boys are twice as frequently affected as girls, but the condition is slightly more common in women than in men

Causes and triggers of asthma

How does asthma start?

Most people know that asthma can 'run in families' and there is undoubtedly a hereditary component to this condition, particularly in allergic (sometimes called extrinsic) asthma.

The genetic factor is much less marked in patients where allergy is not involved (intrinsic asthma).

The tendency to develop asthma is not absolute: it is not inherited in the way that eye colour and blood group are, and a patient with very severe asthma can have children who never develop the condition.

The role of environmental factors (for example, allergens, exposure to passive smoking) are therefore paramount in the development – and exacerbation – of asthma. Nevertheless, it is clear that, in order for the 'seed' of asthma to germinate, the 'soil' must be right!

Factors involved in the initiation of asthma

- Inheritance
- Mother smoking during pregnancy
- Passive smoking in childhood
- Allergens (especially house dust mite)
- 'Colds' or viral infections
- Occupational exposures

House dust mite

Against this background, many factors seem to be responsible for the first appearance of the symptoms of asthma. For instance, asthma beginning in adult life often seems to start following a 'cold' or viral infection; alternatively, exposure to a trigger in the workplace may be the initiating factor.

The most important factor in precipitating asthma, however, part-icularly in children, is exposure to the house dust mite. This little beast, smaller than a pin point, lives in our carpets, mattresses and furry toys. There can be as many as two million in each mattress!

When a susceptible individual is exposed to a protein in the faecal pellet of the mite over a period of time, the body's white cells become sensitive to this 'foreign substance'. As the protein is inhaled, a reaction to it occurs in the lining of the bronchial tubes, resulting in inflammation of the airways. The inflammation makes the lining irritable so that any further exposure, either to the house dust mite or any other potential trigger factor, will result in narrowing of the bronchial tubes and the symptoms of asthma.

There are other factors that contribute to the initiation of asthma. Smoking by the mother during pregnancy and exposure to passive cigarette smoke in childhood may contribute in some cases.

House dust mite.

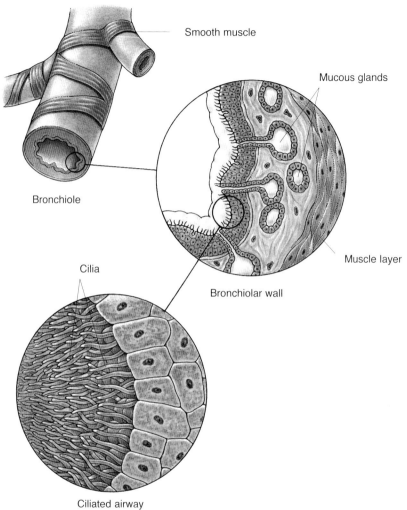

Smooth muscle

Mucous glands

Bronchiole

Muscle layer

Cilia

Bronchiolar wall

Ciliated airway

Anatomy of the airways.

Inflammation and the airways

Asthma, then, is an inflammatory condition, which makes the airways more irritable. Inflammation is the body's attempt to respond to a range of assaults and is seen in many illnesses such as arthritis, colitis and dermatitis. Problems arise for the patient when the inflammation does not resolve and becomes long-standing (or chronic), as is the case in asthma.

The normal airway is lined with a delicate protective layer called the mucosa or epithelium. This layer consists of various types of cell with different jobs. Some can produce mucus, while others help to clear the mucus from the airway by wafting the secretions up the bronchial tubes via movement of tiny fingers or cilia, which are found on the surface of these cells. These cilia are some of the first structures to be destroyed by cigarette smoke, which also stimulates increased mucus production because the smoke causes inflammation. This is the reason why smokers cough up phlegm. In some patients with asthma, cough is also important and this is hardly surprising now we have seen that asthma is an inflammatory condition.

Below the epithelium, a second layer (the submucosa) lies over a spiral sheet of muscle which, in asthma, contracts when a patient inhales a trigger such as grass pollen.

There are three stages in the process leading to airway narrowing and wheezy breathlessness. When the airway becomes inflamed, first of all, the middle layer of the airway becomes swollen; second, the mucous glands produce more secretions (which have to be coughed up to clear the airways); and third, the smooth muscle contracts as a result of release of substances from cells, which appear from the blood in response to an inflammatory trigger or cause.

The net result of these three effects is to narrow the airways, making it more difficult to get air in and out – which leads to wheezy breathlessness. Different forms of treatment have been devised which can attack at each stage of the airway narrowing.

In asthma, symptoms can occur for no obvious reason or may be caused by a clear-cut exposure to a known 'trigger factor' such as grass pollen during the summer. Equally, the airway narrowing can reverse with improvement of symptoms either spontaneously or following the use of a reliever drug. It is this variability that is so characteristic of asthma. We take advantage of this both when making the diagnosis and when devising ways of keeping asthma under control.

Trigger factors in asthma

If you have asthma you will recognise that several factors will set your asthma off.

Exercise

This is a particularly obvious trigger in children, where it may often be the only thing that brings out asthmatic symptoms. The problem is that breathlessness on exertion is often attributed to non-fitness rather than asthma. The schoolboy is then felt to be not fit enough to play as a forward on the football field (putting us in danger of producing a nation of asthmatic goalkeepers!).

CASE HISTORY

John is seven years old and his mother, who had hay fever when younger, had noticed that he had begun to cough when running around in the garden. She had taken him to the GP who had prescribed antibiotics with no benefit on three separate occasions. The symptoms became more persistent and it was only when he developed wheeze on

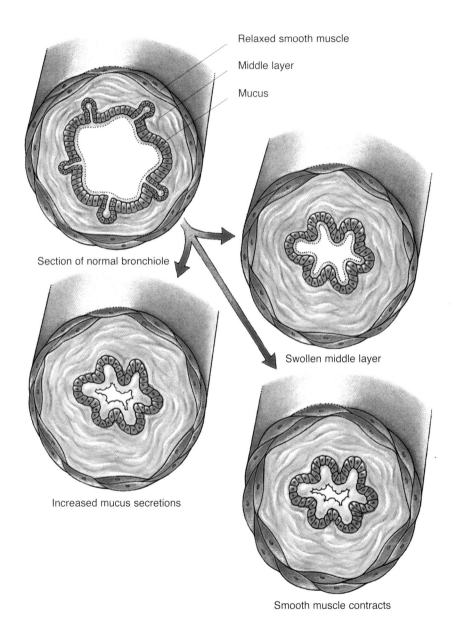

Relaxed smooth muscle

Middle layer

Mucus

Section of normal bronchiole

Swollen middle layer

Increased mucus secretions

Smooth muscle contracts

Changes in the airways during asthma attack.

claims to be able to stroke the cat without 'getting an attack'.

CASE HISTORY

Anne, a 27-year-old woman with long-standing asthma, was referred to a chest physician because of worsening symptoms over the previous two months. She was known to have many allergic triggers for her asthma, including grass and tree pollens and a number of furry animals.

As part of the assessment, the doctor visited her at home to be greeted by 14 cats which, it emerged, she bred and showed, a fact of which her GP was unaware.

exertion during a games lesson at school that the penny dropped and a diagnosis of asthma was made. John was prescribed a bronchodilator (tube opening) inhaler to be used when he has symptoms, since which time he has been well and able to play without getting breathless.

Allergens

Grass pollen is the most frequently recognised allergic trigger but animals, particularly cats and horses, are potent causes of asthma attacks. Chronic exposure to allergens may result in more persistent symptoms, and the importance of animals in the house may be missed as the patient

Trigger factors in asthma

- Exercise
- Inhaled allergens (especially animals)

allergens

exercising

- 'Colds' and viruses
- Fumes/dust/odours

emotions

dust

pollution

- Emotion/stress
- Pollution – indoors and out!
- Cold air
- Foods

Anne had an extremely strong skin test reaction to cat fur but fervently denied that stroking the cats made her worse. It was clear that the cats were a major cause of her continuing asthma, providing a constant exposure to allergen, which effectively gave her recurrent, virtually continuous asthma episodes. She would not get rid of the cats, her best friends, and a balance has had to be struck between bad asthma caused by exposure to allergens and the benefits of keeping her friends and companions.

'Colds' and viruses

Viral infections (common colds) are the commonest trigger for asthma across the age spectrum.

Antibiotics are effective in treating only bacterial infections: viruses are completely unaffected by antibiotics, which have little or no place in the management of asthma yet are consistently prescribed for episodes of worsening asthma.

Fumes, dusts and odours

Cigarette smoke is a potent trigger for many patients, as are dusty environments, where the dust acts as an irritant.

Odours, such as scent or after-shave, can be a trigger for certain individuals but this is not an allergy. Presumably, it is an irritant reaction to the chemicals involved, and the best treatment is avoidance where possible, although this may have important consequences.

CASE HISTORY

Mary had worked for 22 years in the cosmetic department of the local department store. After a viral infection one autumn, she developed asthma which initially proved easy to treat by the usual means. However, over a year she developed worsening symptoms, particularly cough, and the main trigger appeared to be scents. She stopped using perfumes herself but, after an initial slight improvement, her symptoms clearly began to relate to her exposure to perfumes at the store. Eventually she had to give up her job (she was 58) and her symptoms improved immeasurably.

Emotions and stress

Children often become more wheezy at birthday parties, where the combination of excitement and exertion makes asthma more obvious. Asthma was for years regarded as a neurotic condition, but it is now clear that emotional factors act only as triggers, not initiators, of asthma. Excitement, grief and stress can all trigger an asthma attack.

We have occasionally found patients to have attacks when attending funerals and other such stressful situations.

Climate and pollution

Many patients with asthma know that their condition is affected by the weather, but there is no uniform pattern. Some prefer cold to warm weather; others prefer hot, dry atmospheres. You, the patient, know best and will usually adjust your behaviour and treatment accordingly.

Air pollution episodes are well recognised as causing exacerbations of asthma, particularly in patients with more severe asthma, in both the summer ozone periods and the winter episodes.

There is, however, no direct evidence that exposure to air pollution at current levels will turn a non-asthmatic person into an asthmatic patient.

Air pollution episodes are well recognised to cause exacerbations of asthma.

CASE HISTORY

David, a severe asthmatic in his 20s, had had some difficulty in controlling his asthma during the autumn of 1992. He had increased his inhalers and his GP had given him two courses of steroid tablets. Coming up to Christmas, his asthma at last seemed to be stabilising somewhat, when a five-day air pollution episode hit Birmingham, reaching peak levels on Christmas Eve. By that day David's asthma had become very much worse and, in spite of more steroid tablets and increasing use of his nebuliser, he had to be admitted to hospital – a most unacceptable way to spend Christmas!

CASE HISTORY

In June 1994, a severe thunderstorm struck southern Britain, moving from the Southampton area, up through London and then northwards through East Anglia. During this period hundreds of patients presented to casualty departments with attacks of asthma. Many had no idea that they were asthmatic, although most admitted to wheezing with their hay fever (i.e. they had had asthma but had not been told!). It is likely that a specific combination of meteorological factors and high pollen counts was the cause of the outbreak, a rather dramatic example of the weather affecting patients with asthma.

Interacting factors

In many cases, two or more of these factors will interact, and different combinations will be important for different individuals.

Asthma is a very personal condition – what is good for one may not necessarily be good for another, and patterns of avoidance, treatment and planning in advance need to be organised for each individual.

KEY POINTS

✓ Asthma can run in families, but a patient with quite severe asthma can have children who never develop the condition

✓ The most important factor in initiating asthma, particularly in children, is the house dust mite

✓ Symptoms may occur for no obvious reason, or may be caused by exposure to one or more trigger factors, such as exercise, viral infection, fumes and dusts, grief and stress, climate and pollution

✓ Different combinations of trigger factors are important for different patients

Symptoms
and diagnosis

Symptoms

Asthma can present with one or more of four main symptoms: wheeze, breathlessness, cough and chest tightness.

Wheeze and breathlessness are the most well recognised, usually coming on intermittently either in response to a recognised trigger or out of the blue. However, breathlessness without wheeze can frequently occur.

One symptom often not recognised as being caused by asthma is cough – either a dry cough or cough with phlegm – which typically occurs at night or on exercise.

Failure to recognise that cough can be caused by asthma often results in a diagnosis of bronchitis being made. Attacks of bronchitis are usually treated by antibiotics, which is a quite inappropriate treatment for asthma. More than two episodes of persistent cough – with or without wheeze or breathlessness – should raise the question of underlying asthma in the minds of both patient and doctor.

The fourth main symptom of asthma is chest tightness. Often, this occurs on exertion and when this happens in an older patient a diagnosis of angina may be made,

Four main symptoms of asthma

● **Cough**

● **Breathlessness**

● **Chest tightness**

● **Wheeze**

and it may be quite a difficult problem for the doctor to sort out.

Although the symptoms of asthma often occur for no apparent reason, characteristically they can wake patients and are often a problem on waking in the morning. Waking at night with asthma means that the asthma is being inadequately treated. Exercise, particularly in children, is a frequent trigger for worsening symptoms, often resulting in the child missing games at school.

Diagnosis

The trouble with these symptoms is that they occur in many other types of lung – or heart – condition. So, a careful history of what the symptoms are, what sets them off, how long they last, how bad they are and whether there are any recognisable patterns of symptoms, is essential to the doctor in helping him or her arrive at a diagnosis.

Although listening to the chest is part of any examination, very often in asthma it doesn't help the doctor a great deal. The absence of wheezing does NOT mean that asthma isn't the diagnosis!

Conversely, all that wheezes is not asthma – making the diagnosis of asthma not always that easy.

Breathing tests

Although a diagnosis of asthma may have been made on history alone, some simple tests are often used to help.

Conditions that can be confused with asthma

Diagnosis	Wheeze	Breathlessness	Cough	Tightness
Asthma	++	++	++	++
Chronic bronchitis	++	++	++	+
Emphysema	+	++	–	++
Bronchiectasis	+	+	+++	+
Angina	–	+	–	+++
Heart failure	+	++	+	+

Symptom not usually seen   –
Symptom can be seen   +
Symptom often seen   ++
Symptom virtually always seen   +++

ECG or heart trace.

In older patients, in whom heart complaints are common, an electro-cardiogram (ECG or heart trace) may help, but breathing tests form the mainstay of the investigation of asthma.

There are two main types of breathing tests used in diagnosing asthma, each helping in slightly different ways. Both measure how narrow the airways may be, because the narrower the airways, the slower the flow of air through the tubes and the lower the readings.

Peak flow meter

The mini-peak flow meter is small, cheap and robust and gives an idea of the narrowness of the airways by measuring the maximum, or peak rate at which air can be expelled.

This is the method most likely to be used by general practitioners as a single reading in surgery. However, you may be able to use one to

Mini-peak flow meter.

How to use the peak flow meter

1 Stand up if possible

2 Check cursor is on zero (litres/minute or l/min position)

3 Take a deep breath in and place peak flow meter in the mouth (hold horizontally), and close lips

4 Blow suddenly and hard

5 Note number indicated by cursor

6 Return cursor to zero

7 Repeat twice and obtain three readings

8 Write down the best of the three readings

The mini-Wright peak flow meter

If in doubt always seek professional advice

Reproduced by kind permission of the National Asthma & Respiratory Training Centre.

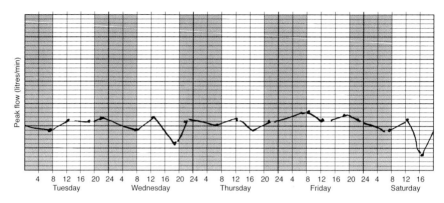

Peak flow chart showing intermittent variation.

Peak flow chart with the common 'morning dip' pattern.

measure your peak flow two, three or four times a day, in order to show variation in values over the day. A normal individual will show very little variation in peak flow over days and weeks, whereas the patient with asthma shows either consistent or intermittent variation.

A common pattern is the 'morning dip' one, values being lowest on waking. Sometimes the fall in peak flow is intermittent, often in response to a recognised trigger such as cat fur. Measuring peak flow in this way is particularly helpful if you complain of only intermittent symptoms.

Measuring lung function using a spirometer.

Daily peak flow monitoring can be extremely helpful in management plans by acting as an 'early warning system' to anticipate worsening asthma.

Spirometry

This is used almost exclusively at chest clinics and in hospitals; it measures not only how fast air can be blown out but also the amount blown out with each breath. It gives us more information but cannot give us the day-to-day measurements of peak flow readings.

'Reversibility' tests

Sometimes these breathing tests are performed before and after inhalation of a bronchodilator drug, which opens the tubes. If the readings increase by 15 per cent or more after inhaling the drug, the airway narrowing is said to be reversible and confirms a diagnosis of asthma. Even asthmatic patients do not always show reversibility on every occasion tested, but it is nevertheless a very useful diagnostic test in patients in whom asthma is suspected.

Other breathing tests

If your diagnosis is difficult to sort out, you may be sent to a lung function laboratory; here more complicated tests are arranged, usually at the request of a hospital doctor.

KEY POINTS

✓ The four main symptoms of asthma are wheeze, breathlessness, cough and chest tightness

✓ Waking at night with asthma means that the asthma is being inadequately treated

✓ More than two episodes of persistent cough should suggest asthma

✓ All that wheezes is not asthma, and the absence of wheezing doesn't mean that asthma is not the diagnosis

Prevention and self-help

Although a diagnosis of asthma may seem to lead inevitably to the use of drugs to control the condition, there are several ways in which you and your family can help reduce symptoms. Equally, there are some environmental modifications that are not believed to be of help.

Avoiding allergens

Controlling the house dust mite can be very important in some patients, but the measures are expensive. Occlusive bedding is effective but extremely costly unless simple polythene sheeting is used completely to enclose the mattress and each pillow. This makes for a very crinkly and sweaty bed, however! Sprays to kill the mites are ineffective on their own in controlling asthma. In theory, carpets and loose fittings should be removed and some recommend blinds instead of curtains. Cuddly

Helping yourself or helping your child

- Don't smoke cigarettes
- Avoid 'colds' where possible
- Control allergen exposures
- Establish a self-management plan with the help of your doctor

- Keep teachers informed about your child's asthma and the need for access to inhalers on demand
- Where obvious triggers are known – avoid them!

toys should be put in the deep freeze for 12 hours a week to kill the mites. Because these measures are time-consuming or expensive, inhaled therapy is a much easier method of controlling symptoms for most people.

Getting rid of domestic pets is a contentious issue. Where there is undoubted allergy to cats, dogs or rabbits, a balance has to be struck between control of asthma using inhalers and the grief that can be caused by banishing the pet! Nevertheless, long-term exposure to pets, even those that do not induce an obvious attack, can chronically worsen asthma by exposing a sensitised patient to high levels of allergen. In the more severe asthmatic patient, where control is more difficult, sometimes we have to insist on removal.

I believe that patients' wishes are very important. Some would rather get rid of a pet than use inhalers; others would rather suffer asthma than lose what is often their best friend. Only when beliefs and wishes cause risk to the patient should we be emphatic about parting with the pet.

Central heating

There is no direct evidence one way or the other that any particular form of central heating is either good or bad for patients with asthma. The belief that gas fired central heating dries the air too much has been reported by some patients with asthma, but it is unlikely that this is a major problem. On the other hand, there is good reason to believe that ducted or warm air central heating may cause a problem, especially in those patients with allergy to house dust mite. Unfortunately, it is extremely expensive to replace such systems, especially when there is no guarantee that the patient will improve after removal. I do, however, advise my patients to avoid installing these systems if they are putting in a new one.

Bedroom temperature

A famous doctor of the seventeenth century, Sir John Floyer, himself an asthmatic, believed that when asthma woke a patient up at night this was due to 'the heat of the bed'! Equally, it has been said that sleeping with the bedroom window open, or at least keeping the air cool at night is a help to asthmatics. In truth, there is no clear-cut answer. Some prefer the cooler night air, others will find it causes them to wheeze more, particularly if they have to get up at night for some other reason. Again, it is up to you to adjust your environment according to what suits you best.

Viral infections

Viruses are an unavoidable cause of worsening asthma but it makes sense to put off a visit to or from someone with a streaming cold! For mums and schoolchildren, however, this is unavoidable – children have to go to school and should not be kept off just because of the risk of catching a cold.

Diet

A small proportion of patients with asthma, particularly children, undoubtedly have food sensitivities. Again, a balance has to be struck between the wishes of the patient and control of asthma.

True food allergy is not particularly common but is undoubtedly more common than many doctors believe. The diagnosis is often difficult and involves time-consuming tests. In an important minority, identifying a food or foods that worsen an individual's asthma can have a dramatic effect. A clear history of, for example, wheezing within minutes of eating a peanut, is easy to recognize, and the best treatment is avoidance. On the other hand, sensitivity to dairy products or wheat is more difficult to recognise because the effects are more chronic and not so dramatic.

CASE HISTORY

Nick had had asthma since childhood and he had always known that peanuts made him worse and could cause very severe attacks. He had managed this by scrupulously avoiding all peanut-containing foods, often a difficult job! During his teens his asthma improved considerably but he still avoided peanuts. On the odd occasion when he took in a mouthful of food containing peanuts he would immediately notice a tingling sensation in his mouth and would spit out the uneaten food. This usually prevented an attack.

One day, while eating a meal at the house of his new girl friend, he suddenly realised that he had swallowed a mouthful of peanut-containing food. Within minutes, his tongue and lips had swollen and he had begun a severe asthma attack.

By the time he reached hospital he was blue and unconscious. Luckily, he had been got there extremely quickly but he still required ventilation for a short period before recovering. His girl friend and her mother were mortified as they had been unaware of his peanut allergy – one of the food allergies that patients rarely if ever grow out of – thus highlighting the dangers of 'hidden' food allergens.

If you think you are sensitive to certain foods, you should be investigated by a doctor with relevant expertise.

CASE HISTORY

Carolyn was 35 years old and had had asthma since her teens. Initially, it had affected her quality of life but she had managed to develop a career and generally had her asthma under good control. Over a period of two to three years, however, she began to suffer worsening symptoms and found she was needing frequent courses of oral steroids. Concerned, she asked to be referred to hospital where drug treatment was increased to a maximum without success. She was then admitted to hospital to undergo a food exclusion regimen, which suggested that she might be sensitive to wheat products. When challenged with wheat in capsule form after a period of abstension, her asthma deteriorated over a week, confirming the suspicion. Since avoiding wheat her asthma has been well controlled, although she is still on inhalers at moderate dose, and she has only rarely needed a course of oral steroids.

If you are shown to have a problem, avoiding the foods is the only way forward. For foods that are not often eaten (for example, shellfish) avoidance is relatively straight-forward. However, if you are sensitive to dairy products or wheat – two of the more common recognised problem foodstuffs – the diet may become particularly tiresome and antisocial, especially if your asthma symptoms are modest. Some patients would rather stick to a diet than take any drugs at all. Only rarely will asthma symptoms be completely controlled by dietary means, which should be seen as complementary to adequate medical treatment.

Cigarette smoke

Cigarette smoke is bad for asthma. Sadly, 15 to 20 per cent of patients

Cigarette smoke is bad for asthma.

with asthma smoke and these patients are more likely to end up in hospital with acute asthma and to develop irreversible narrowing of their airways. If you smoke, you must try to stop by whatever means you

Smoking during pregnancy increases the chance of the child being born with asthma.

can – this requires a great deal of help from relatives and friends. 'Just the one' will hurt, and offering you a cigarette is a far from friendly act.

Inhaling other people's second-hand smoke (passive smoking) causes considerable suffering to children with asthma. The children of parents who smoke are more likely to have wheezy episodes and time off school than are children with non-smoking parents. This is most marked when both parents smoke, but maternal smoking seems to be more of a problem than father's smoke because children usually spend more time with their mums.

Smoking during pregnancy increases the risk of the child being born with asthma, even allowing for all other risk factors such as family history.

Games and school

Exercise-induced asthma is common in children and can cause problems, with teachers accusing kids of 'not trying' or attempting to avoid games lessons, and their own school mates teasing them for 'being useless' and other such colourful taunts. Sensible preparation can help. It is always a good idea for an asthmatic child to take either a relief inhaler or Intal about 15 minutes before going out to play games. If it is used just as he

runs on to the pitch, symptoms will develop before the inhaler has a chance to work.

In some children, after the first episode of wheezing with exercise, there often follows a period when they can run long and hard without problems, which may last for the rest of the session. This so-called 'refractory period' sometimes, unfortunately, has the effect of reinforcing to a sceptical teacher or schoolmate that the child was always trying to 'skive'!

This brings up the whole subject of asthma in school. Many teachers are somewhat uninformed about asthma, although it must be said that they are very keen to know more if offered the chance. If you have an asthmatic child, you should take the opportunity to tell your child's teachers about the need for your son or daughter to have ready access to a relief inhaler. All too often we hear of inhalers being locked away in the school secretary's office, which may be some distance from the school playing field. By explaining to the teachers how to allow the use of a relief inhaler without permitting its abuse, the teacher's worries about the perceived dangers of inhalers will be dispelled.

Athletes and asthma

Many top sportsmen and sportswomen have asthma and are able to compete at the highest level. Some of the self-help advice given above for children is applicable to adults, particularly as far as use of inhalers before exertion is concerned. A warm-up period will also help to some extent with the problem of exercise-induced symptoms when doing the first exercise of the day.

KEY POINTS

✓ Controlling the house dust mite is important for some patients but expensive to achieve

✓ Ducted or warm air central heating may cause a problem, especially in patients allergic to the house dust mite

✓ Severe asthma may necessitate parting with a pet

✓ Patients with food allergy can rarely control their asthma symptoms by dietary means only

✓ Asthmatic patients who smoke must stop

✓ Smoking during pregnancy increases the risk of the child being born with asthma

✓ Parents of an asthmatic child may need to explain to teachers the need for their child to have ready access to his or her relief inhaler

✓ For a sportsman or sportswoman, a warm-up period before doing the first exercise of the day will help ameliorate exercise-induced symptoms

Drugs used in the treatment of asthma

The drugs used for the treatment of asthma can be divided into three main groups: relievers, preventers and emergency or reserve drugs.

Categories of drugs used to treat asthma

- Relievers
- Preventers
- Emergency/reserve drugs

Relievers

These drugs act by relaxing the muscle in the walls of the airways, allowing the airway to open up and air to get in and out more easily. The result is that breathing is eased. These are called bronchodilator drugs and are given in inhaled form, the inhaler usually being blue or grey in colour. Inhalers come in a range of different types of inhaler device. In most cases, inhalers should be used when symptoms occur rather than on

Drugs used in the treatment of asthma

Normal   Asthma attack

Acting on smooth muscle in
the wall of the airway

'Reliever' drugs act by relaxing the muscle in the walls of the airways, allowing
the airway to open up.

a regular basis, although if you have more severe asthma, regular use may be needed on the advice of your doctor.

Preventers

These drugs act by reducing the inflammation in the airways, thus calming their irritability. In contrast to reliever inhalers, they must be taken on a regular basis, usually twice a day. In a way, they are like a toothbrush – regular use will keep you out of trouble! Indeed, many patients keep their preventer inhaler next to their toothbrush as a reminder, as it is sometimes easy to forget to take the preventer inhaler when asthma is well controlled and symptoms few and far between.

Main types of preventer drugs

Type of drug	Delivery method
Inhaled steroids	Inhaled
Cromoglycate – Intal	Inhaled
Nedocromil – Tilade	Inhaled
Theophylline preparations	Tablets

There are three main types of preventer drugs: inhaled steroids, cromoglycate (Intal) and nedocromil (Tilade). Again, these come in a variety of different inhaler devices (see page 48).

Inhaled steroids

The word 'steroid' conjures up disturbing pictures in many people's minds, and there is much mis-information circulating about these very effective drugs.

- These steroids are **not** the anabolic steroids used by bodybuilders and illegally by some athletes.
- The inhaled version used as preventive treatment **is** the same sort of drug as tablet steroids used for acute attacks of asthma and, for example, in some patients with arthritis.
- The dose of the inhaled drug is extremely **small** compared with that contained in steroid tablets. For instance, two puffs twice a day from a Becotide 100 inhaler delivers 400 micrograms of drug. In acute asthma, six 5 milligram (mg) tablets will be given per day – 30,000 micrograms of drug, 75 times the dose.
- The side-effects of inhaled steroids are few compared with

Drugs used in the treatment of asthma

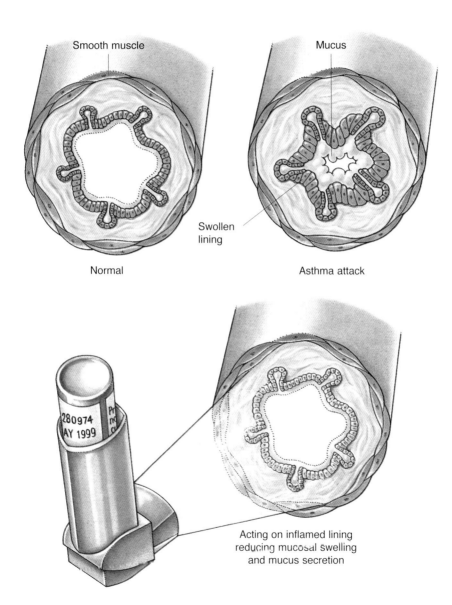

Smooth muscle

Mucus

Swollen lining

Normal

Asthma attack

Acting on inflamed lining reducing mucosal swelling and mucus secretion

'Preventer' drugs act by reducing the inflammation in the airways, thus calming their irritability.

those of oral steroids but, **most importantly**, are very much less than the dangers of undertreated asthma.

- Four per cent of patients on inhaled steroids will complain of a sore or dry mouth (sometimes this is due to thrush) while a further 4 per cent may complain of some huskiness of voice; this is more important for some patients who use their voice a lot (such as teachers or telephone operators) than for others.
- At higher doses (1,500 micrograms per day or more), particularly in older patients, side-effects, such as easy bruising, may become apparent along with an increase in the frequency of oral thrush and hoarseness. Cataracts may occur in some patients but the suggestion that inhaled steroids cause osteoporosis (thinning of the bones) is debatable. Any such effects have to be balanced against the risks of undertreated asthma. The local effects of these inhalers can be minimised by mouth-washing after each dose and by use of large volume spacer devices (see later) which act as 'reservoirs' and markedly reduce the amount of drug deposited in the mouth.

- There is some evidence that in high doses a small proportion of children may show slight growth suppression with inhaled steroids but, interestingly, once the asthmatic child reaches adult height, growth catch-up has virtually always occurred.

Chronic, undertreated asthma of childhood is more likely to cause growth suppression than are inhaled steroids.

Inhaled steroids are very effective preventive drugs across the full spectrum of patients with asthma and are regarded as the preventive treatment of choice in most patients with asthma.

Cromoglycate (Intal)

Sodium cromoglycate has been available for as long as inhaled steroids. It is a very good form of prevention in the milder forms of childhood asthma, particularly in controlling exercise-induced symptoms. It needs to be used three or four times a day, a disadvantage when compared with inhaled steroids, but it can be used simply before exercise to prevent exercise-induced symptoms and has virtually no side-effects.

44

Types of inhaled drugs

RELIEVERS		PREVENTERS	
Drug name	**Inhaler name**	**Drug name**	**Inhaler name**
Salbutamol	Ventolin (inc. Ventidisks)	Beclomethasone	Becotide 50; 100; 200 micrograms (inc. Becodisks)
	Salbulin Salamol Aerolin		Becloforte Beclazone series AeroBec series Filair series
Terbutaline	Bricanyl (inc. Turbohaler)	Budesonide	Pulmicort 100, 200, 480 micrograms (inc. Turbohaler)
Fenoterol	Berotec	Fluticasone	Flixotide 25; 50; 125; 250 micrograms (inc. Diskhaler series)
Salmeterol	Serevent	Cromoglycate	Intal (puffer 5 micrograms) (spincaps 20 micrograms)
Eformoterol	Foradil		Cromogen
Ipratropium	Atrovent Atrovent forte	Nedocromil	Tilade
Oxitropium	Oxivent	Beclomethasone & salbutamol	Ventide
Fenoterol & ipratropium	Duovent	Cromoglycate & salbutamol	Aerocrom
Salbutamol & ipratropium	Combivent		

Nedocromil (Tilade)

Nedocromil sodium has a preventive strength similar to that of low-dose inhaled steroids and comes as a mint-flavoured dry powder aerosol.

Theophylline preparations

Also to be included under preventive treatment is the group of tablets known collectively as the theophyllines (for example, Uniphyllin, Phyllocontin, Nuelin, Theodur). These were originally used as bronchodilators but tend to be used more in a preventive way now. They are probably used less than in the past because of the effectiveness and safety of inhaled steroids. They tend to cause nausea and headache in some patients but have the advantage of being something you just swallow – some people have difficulty mastering the use of an inhaler.

Emergency or reserve treatment

When an acute attack of asthma occurs there are two mainstays of emergency treatment available:

1. Big doses of *reliever drug* are given (often via a nebuliser).
2. Big doses of an *anti-inflammatory* drug (injected or oral steroids) are given.

Some patients will be able to self-start emergency treatment with a nebuliser and/or a course of tablet steroids, but for most patients who have not had a severe attack before, they should contact their GP as quickly as possible or attend the local casualty department. Delay can be very dangerous and it is better to be safe than sorry.

Nebulised drugs used in acute episodes are salbutamol (Ventolin), terbutaline (Bricanyl) or ipratropium (Atrovent). Nebulisers should only be obtained after assessment by your doctor. The machine itself is a simple air compressor, which bubbles air through a solution of the drug

The nebuliser is a simple air compressor. It bubbles air through a solution of the drug, generating a mist which is inhaled through either a mask or a mouthpiece.

generating a mist which is inhaled through either a mask or a mouthpiece. The compressors themselves are not always available through the NHS in every health district. You may have to buy your own or obtain one, often on a loan basis, through a charity such as the National Asthma Campaign (see page 91), whose local branches often run a nebuliser loan service.

Sometimes, nebulised drugs are prescribed to be used regularly in the more severe patient but only when high doses of other treatments have proved inadequate. Nebulisers should not be used as an alternative to inhaled preventive treatment.

Delivery devices

In many patients the simple metered dose inhalers (puffers) just cannot be used effectively. Poor inhaler technique can result in all the drug escaping into the air through the top of the inhaler.

The patient then believes that the inhaler is 'no good' whereas it is not being given half a chance to work. If you are one of these patients, you can use another type of inhaler device that relies on your breath in sucking the drug into the lung, as opposed to the puffer, where breathing in has to coincide with the squirt of the puffer.

The most frequently used type of 'breath-activated' device is the spacer where the spacer acts as a reservoir of drug from the puffer for the patient then to breathe in at the right moment. Spacers are made of brittle plastic and there is some evidence that they acquire quite a lot of static electrical charge, which makes the drug stick to the inside of the spacer, thus reducing the amount of drug getting into the lungs. The best plan is to wash the spacer once a week and allow it to drip dry. Rubbing with an anti-static cloth, such as can be found in Hi-Fi shops, can also help

The range of inhaler devices (not drawn to scale).

reduce this problem. Other types of breath-activated devices are Rota-halers, Turbohalers, Diskhalers and Autohalers, all of which have their benefits and shortcomings. In many cases it is clear that an individual patient is very much at home with a particular device.

Matching the patient with the right device is vital, as an acceptable device is more likely to be used at the right time and effectively. With the exception of the spacer devices, 'breath-activated devices' are more expensive, although a correctly used 'expensive' device may, in the long term, be cheaper in terms of patient suffering than a poorly used 'cheap' device.

KEY POINTS

✓ Drugs used in asthma treatment are either relievers, preventers or emergency (reserve) drugs

✓ Inhaled steroids are the preventive treatment of choice in most patients with asthma

✓ In an emergency, patients who have not had a severe attack before should contact their GP as quickly as possible or attend the local casualty department. Delay can be very dangerous

✓ Nebulisers should not be used as an alternative to inhaled preventive treatment

Management – patient, doctor and nurse

The whole aim of managing asthma is to put you, the patient, in control of your asthma rather than have the asthma being in control of you. In patients who require only the occasional puff of their relief inhaler, this is straightforward, but for patients with more significant asthma, guidelines – or battle plans – need to be devel- oped and agreed by doctor and patient.

Although we have already said that asthma is a very personal condition and that what is right for one may not be right for another, there are, nevertheless, guidelines that have recently been developed to help nurses and doctors in the management of all their asthmatic patients. These were developed by a panel of experts representing the different groups involved in the management of asthma.

The guidelines are simple to use but have not yet been taken up by as many doctors as we would like. They are based on a series of upward steps in treatment to control asthma and a series of downward steps when asthma appears to be in good control and when lower doses of treatment may be possible.

Before I describe the steps, just let me remind you about the importance of preventive measures, similar to those discussed in the Self-help section on page 29, which include control of allergens. It is very important to avoid certain drugs that cause asthma or make it worse (for example, aspirin, beta-blockers). Even if you have been taking these medications for some time without problems, if you begin to develop wheezy breathlessness, stop taking these tablets. You should also stop drugs similar to aspirin, and seek alternatives (see section on Special forms of asthma on page 63).

Guideline steps

Step 1

Most patients fit into this level. Patients are advised to use their relief inhaler as required. If you are using it regularly more than once a day, you will move to Step 2. If your use of the relief inhaler stays at less than one puff a day on average, no further drug treatment need be considered, although if your relief inhaler use increases you must see your doctor.

Step 2

If you are using more than one puff a day of relief inhaler on average, you need a preventive inhaler, the choice of which is made by the doctor as a general rule (see section on Drugs used in the treatment of asthma, page 40). This should result in you reducing the use of an inhaled reliever to less than one puff a day.

Step 3

If your symptoms persist, your doctor will start you on higher doses of inhaled preventive treatment or consider a different preventive drug. Again, these decisions need to be made by the doctor but in discussion with you, the patient, and after assessment of your particular needs.

Subsequent steps

If you are still having problems the use of even higher doses of inhaled preventive treatment, oral steroid use and nebulisers, among other treatment options, will be considered. At this stage, or at Step 3, it is likely that you will be referred to a chest consultant for assessment, but we like to think that up to this step you will be managed by your general practitioner.

Step down

In medicine it is sometimes perhaps too easy to start a new treatment when symptoms do not come under control. It is not so easy to stop a treatment either because symptoms are well controlled or because the new drug had no extra benefit.

The guidelines suggest ways of carefully reducing treatment in patients who are well controlled without losing the ground gained.

Management plans

One way of giving you particularly good control over your asthma and its treatment is to provide you with a management plan. This is a series of instructions on what to do when your asthma starts to slip or in situations in which your asthma may be thought likely to worsen.

There are two types of management plan.

Peak flow-based management plans

The peak flow meter is simple to use and to read. A short sharp blow will record the maximum rate at which air can be blown out of your lungs. Usually, three attempts are

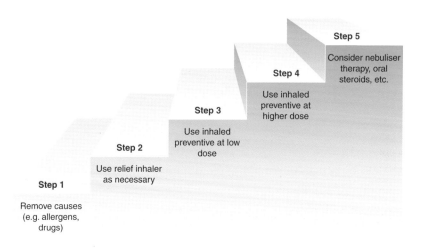

Stepwise approach to the control of asthma.

made, and you record the highest. Recording a value twice a day (on waking and on going to bed) is usually sufficient although sometimes the doctor will ask for more frequent recordings.

With a peak flow-based management plan you will be provided with a peak flow meter, a chart on which to record the peak flow readings, along with two target values.

The first level is the **target peak flow**, which is usually about 70 per cent of best. If your peak flow is above this value, you need not adjust your treatment, but if your peak flow falls below this over a 24-hour period, you should double your

---

DATE THIS CARD WAS STARTED:

ASK YOUR DOCTOR TO FILL THIS IN FOR YOU.

BAD ATTACK
WHAT TO LOOK FOR:

● Very tight chest, hard to breathe.

● Too wheezy to walk or talk properly.

● Your reliever inhaler does not help your breathing.

● Peak flow under
and does not go up after taking your reliever inhaler.

WHAT TO DO:

● Take

● and take   mg.

(tablets)

AT THE SAME TIME: please tick
● Call your doctor

● Dial 999

● Go to the nearest hospital

TAKE THIS CARD WITH YOU
WHENEVER YOU SEE YOUR DOCTOR.

INSTRUCTIONS
Be sure to fill in the record card every day
Section 1.
Record your daily symptoms by ticking if present in the relevant section.
Section 2.
Record your peak flow by using your peak flow meter in the morning and evening. Mark a cross on the graph against the score for the best of three blows.

Section 3.
Write down in the boxes next to the treatments you take the number of times you take the medicine in 24 hours.

WK 1	MON	TUE
a.		
b.	✓	
c.		✓
d.		
e.	✓	

	AM	PM	AM	PM
700				
650				
600				
550				
500				
450				
400				
350				
300				
250				
200				
150				
100				
50				

1	2	2
2	2	2
3		
4		
5		

Peak flow chart used in management plans.

inhaled preventive treatment until your peak flows have climbed above the target peak flow.

The second value is usually about 50 per cent of best. At this level you should use a course of oral steroids, only if the double dose of inhaled preventive has not worked. You may be allowed to take this course of action yourself, although some doctors prefer to see the patient if oral steroids are needed. A final threshold is that at which you should seek medical assistance as soon as possible, from either your GP or the local casualty department. This level of peak flow will be set by the doctor.

The chart for recording peak flows may either be a series of columns on which the recordings are written, usually twice a day, or a graph-like chart to plot the values. Some patients prefer this second form of chart because the variation in levels of peak flow can be more easily appreciated.

CASE HISTORY

William had always been a difficult little lad, and not just as far as his asthma was concerned. He tended to take his inhalers only when he felt the need and consequently was constantly missing school. By the time he had reached secondary school, with no sign of his asthma abating, his GP decided to try and establish a management plan. For the first time William started to record his peak flow readings at home on waking and on going to bed. The peak flow meter stayed by his bed and his parents were able to check that he was recording the values on his chart. Somewhat to his surprise, William found that his peak flow readings varied considerably, dropping as low as 150 on waking but reaching 270 by evening time.

The penny having dropped, he began to take his inhaled preventive more regularly and the peak flow variation became less marked, the readings also increasing somewhat to settle between 300 and 350. By that stage he was taking two puffs at night and morning of inhaled Becotide 100 and had begun to use the relief inhaler much less frequently. The GP then gave him a target peak flow of 275, advising him to double his Becotide if the values dropped below this over a 24-hour period and keeping at the higher dose until he was above target for at least three days.

A second threshold was given of 175, below which William knew to contact his GP for a course of oral steroids. In the event, oral steroids did not become necessary. William began to notice the benefits of his regular preventive therapy and over the subsequent year had to increase his inhaled steroids (peak flows fell below 275) on only three occasions.

Symptom-based management plans

The same concept as that of a peak flow-based plan operates here except that certain levels of symptoms are used as prompts for changes in treatment as opposed to changes in peak flow.

CASE HISTORY

Jacky had not got on well with peak flow measurements. They did not seem to tell her much more about her asthma than did her symptoms and they began to be a pain to do, being 'just for the sake of the doctor', as she saw it. Luckily, the GP became aware of this and suggested a switch to a symptom-based plan. By doubling her inhaled preventive if she used more than three puffs of relief inhaler a day over two successive days, or when she started a cold, or if she started to wake at night with symptoms, her asthma was more effectively controlled. If doubling the inhaled preventive didn't stop her symptoms she knew she had to go to her GP for reassessment, although if she had to do that she did measure her peak flow a few times before the consultation 'just to see'. This helped the GP believe that she was managing her asthma sensibly.

Choosing a plan

Some patients seem better suited to peak flow-based plans, others to symptom-based plans, and the decision which to use is often based on a number of factors. Sometimes a combination of symptoms and peak flow can be used for certain individuals. Both types of plan will include advice to anticipate problems such as colds or exposure to known allergens. If you develop the early symptoms of a cold (runny nose etc.) you should double your inhaled preventive treatment and continue for at least a week until the cold and its effects have passed, when you can resume the original dose. Some patients only need inhaled steroids for colds and they should start at the slightest beginnings of a cold and continue for two weeks unless their asthma still continues to cause problems, in which case they should stay on their preventive treatment and contact their GP.

Clinic nurses

Recently, asthma clinics have been set up in many GP surgeries, run either by the general practitioner or by the practice nurse. Some of these clinics do little more than check inhaler technique but the better ones are run by nurses who have been specifically trained in the management of asthma at recognised training centres. Their role in the management of asthma is very important and they have helped provide a much better service for the asthmatic patient in general practice, with fewer referrals to hospital from practices where such a system operates and more appropriate referrals when the patient is running into problems.

Often, the asthma nurse will see patients with asthma more than the doctor will, releasing the doctor for other patients, but the nurse knows very well when the doctor needs to see the patient if things are not going well. It ought to be the aim of all general practices to set up an asthma clinic run by a fully trained asthma nurse.

KEY POINTS

✓ Guidelines have been developed to help nurses and doctors provide optimal management of all asthmatic patients

✓ Many GP surgeries have set up asthma clinics, often run by specially trained asthma nurses

✓ One way of giving patients good control over their asthma is to provide them with management plans

✓ Management plans may either be peak flow based or symptom based

Asthma in elderly people

Asthma tends to be regarded as a condition of the young, particularly children, and indeed it is very much more common in children, as we have seen. As these patients become older, some have persistent symptoms, some have only minor symptoms and some have shed their symptoms to all intents and purposes.

But there are also patients who develop asthma for the first time in their later years, often to their great irritation. It is often believed that these patients are more likely to have more severe asthma and to have to take oral steroids. It is also believed that allergies are less likely to be found. While these beliefs are true up to a point, it is important to realise that there is always a great overlap in patterns of asthma throughout the ages. Yet again, it bears repeating that each patient needs to be assessed as an individual.

Symptoms

The symptoms in the older patient

are identical to those in the younger patient with asthma except that breathlessness, especially on exertion, is quite common. This is often due to the fact that many folk over the age of 60 have, at some stage, smoked cigarettes and are left with a bit of irreversible bronchial tube narrowing. This means that exertion will cause breathlessness more quickly in some individuals.

Where problems can occur is when an older patient complains of chest tightness on exertion. As heart disease is common in this age group and angina can cause this very same symptom, delay in diagnosis – both of angina and asthma – can occur.

CASE HISTORY

An 82-year-old man went to his GP with a six-month history of episodes of breathlessness. Sometimes these came on out of the blue and sometimes when he exerted himself. He did not feel that he was wheezy but did admit that he got a tight feeling in his chest, particularly when he got breathless on exertion.

Quite rightly, the GP's first impression in a gentleman of this age was that this was likely to be due to heart disease, but treatment for angina had no effect. He was sent to a consultant at hospital who felt that late-onset asthma needed to be ruled out, although he was fairly certain that this was an unlikely diagnosis. To the consultant's surprise and delight, the peak flow readings recorded assiduously by the patient showed the typical variation seen in asthma, and prescription of anti-asthma medication resulted in great improvements in his symptoms.

The patient's reaction on realising he had asthma was interesting in that his major reaction was one of anger.

'Why me? I've never smoked and always looked after myself. There's no one in the family who has suffered from asthma. Why me?'

Explanation and reassurance and the fact that on two puffs twice a day of inhaled steroid he improved greatly did relieve his anger. He is now able to garden as he did before with only occasional need to use his relief inhaler.

Treatment

Again, treatment of asthma in the older patient with asthma is the same, and follows the same steps, as in the younger patient. Where problems can occur is in the manageability of the inhaler devices. The Rotacap dry powder system can be very fiddly for an arthritic hand and even the metered dose inhaler (puffer) can be impossible to use by patients with stiff or painful hands. Attachments are available to make the puffer usable by these patients (Haleraid, made by Allen & Hanburys and available on request from chemists), but often the simple expedient of a large volume spacer will ease the problem. It is really a matter of tailoring the inhaler device to the patient.

As age creeps up, patients often find themselves on a variety of different pills, potions and other medications for a range of con-ditions. This can often be very confusing and it is incumbent on the doctor to keep the 'regimen' of treatment as simple as possible. It may even be necessary to sacrifice the ideal treatment just to ensure that the most important treatments are taken.

Side-effects of any form of treat-ment are more common in the older patient. In the more severe asthmatic the side-effects of oral steroids can be severe, particularly the skin changes, with easy bruising, skin thinning and poor wound healing. Patients taking high-dose inhaled steroids (more than 1,500 micrograms per day) can also develop these skin changes, although to a less dramatic degree.

Outlook

Asthma starting in later years is unlikely to leave the patient, who usually has found an unwanted companion for life. The severity does not necessarily get worse, however, and good treatment properly applied will be very effective in controlling symptoms.

Each individual will have his or her own targets or needs. For some it will simply be the ability to potter in the garden, which their untreated asthma may have stopped them doing. Others may wish to be able to go rambling again, or to be able to do their own shopping or go to the pub for a drink with their friends. Success is achieving their own target, not necessarily increasing the dose of inhaler up and up to try and achieve an improvement that the patient may not want or need.

As I mentioned earlier, deaths from asthma have increased in elderly people over the past five to ten years, but the reasons for this are not clear. I suspect that many would have been regarded as having died of bronchitis in days gone by, but we must not be complacent in our attempts to prevent death from asthma at whatever age it may be causing problems.

The outlook for the older patient with asthma should be regarded positively. The treatment is safe and effective although the more severe patient may need to find a balance between symptoms of asthma and side-effects of drugs.

KEY POINTS

✓ Asthma can develop later in life, and these sufferers are more prone to breathlessness, especially on exertion

✓ Angina and asthma in elderly people can be difficult to differentiate

✓ Side-effects of asthma treatment are more common in older patients

✓ Although the asthma is unlikely to go away, elderly sufferers can enjoy effective control of their symptoms with proper treatment targeted to their individual needs

Special forms of asthma

Allergic asthma

If an allergy, or more than one allergy, has been identified as being potentially important on the basis of your history, it is sometimes necessary to do further tests to confirm this and to identify the allergen. The test is simple and takes about half an hour to complete.

A series of drops of various solutions of substances, which are known to cause allergic reactions (for example, house dust mite, grass pollen, tree pollen, cat, etc.), are placed on the forearm. Using small needle points, the skin surface is then gently pierced through each droplet to allow the substance to get under the skin. After 15 minutes or so, local reactions can occur, which look like small areas of nettle rash and usually itch. The needle pricks themselves are not painful – just a tiny scratch – but the itching can be maddening and lasts half an hour or so.

The size of the reaction (or weal) can be measured for each allergen, which gives an idea, not only of what

Food products

Pet dander

House dust mite

Feathers

Pollen

Washing powder

Allergens come in many shapes and sizes; these are just a few!

you are allergic to, but also how allergic you may be to each allergen. Sometimes this is helpful in management because it could tell you which triggers to avoid and could identify things which may turn out to be not so important.

The danger is that small reactions may not be important and patients take unnecessary actions. I have seen the occasional patient on extraordinary and unnecessary diets, based on weakly positive skin tests, which have not helped their asthma. This is not always the case: everyone is an individual and his or her needs must be individually addressed.

Desensitisation

If you are shown to be allergic to a particular allergen (for example, cat or rabbit), if you can't avoid contact with these animals, and your asthma continues to be poorly controlled by the usual treatment regimens, desensitisation may be considered. This should only be done at specialist centres and in my opinion should only be undertaken for one allergen at a time. Certainly for patients with asthma they should be conducted only at a hospital because there have been many examples of severe reactions to desensitisation, with attacks of asthma needing hospital admission and even deaths. For hay fever alone the dangers are less, but for asthma great care needs to be taken.

The process involves a series of injections of small amounts of the substance to which you are allergic, usually under the skin of the upper arm. Very, very small quantities are used to start with, the concentrations increasing week by week to avoid severe allergic reactions. There are different time-scales over which the courses of injections are undertaken before a course is considered complete and this will be up to the centre involved and your needs. Small local reactions (a reddening of the skin at the injection site) are not infrequent but these settle quickly on the day of the injection. Once the course is complete, boosters can be given at varying intervals if the course has been thought successful.

In the UK, desensitisation for asthma is only rarely undertaken, largely because of the fear of bad reactions, but also because many doctors do not believe that this treatment works. If you wish to talk further about whether this might be of use (and it is likely to be useful in only a minority of patients with asthma), then ask your GP for a referral to a centre with experience in this area. A list of specialist centres can be obtained from the British

Allergy Foundation (see Useful addresses on page 91).

Brittle asthma

Brittle asthma is a rare form of asthma. The patient suffers from sudden severe attacks, sometimes in spite of apparently being very well controlled. Others develop attacks on a background of asthma, which doctor and patient have great difficulty in controlling on a day-to-day basis. These patients keep being admitted to hospital and are at increased risk of dying from their asthma.

Allergy seems to be more common in these patients and sometimes their acute attacks follow inhaling or eating something to which they are allergic.

If you are unsure whether a particular drug might interfere with your asthma, ask your GP or your pharmacist

Their asthma often puts a huge strain on both the patient and family, and psychological factors seem to be very important – but whether the asthma causes the psychological disturbance or the other way around is a moot point.

Treatment is extremely difficult and patients should be managed by chest specialists with an interest in the severer forms of asthma.

Aspirin-sensitive asthma

Aspirin sensitivity occurs in around 5 per cent of patients with asthma. It is more common in adults than in children. Very often these patients are negative on skin testing for allergens and may suffer from nasal polyps on a recurring basis. If you are such a patient you must avoid all aspirin-containing drugs, including a wide range of arthritis drugs such as ibuprofen, diclofenac and indomethacin. If you are unsure whether a particular drug might interfere with your asthma, ask your GP or your pharmacist. Aspirin-sensitive asthmatic patients can die from unwittingly swallowing a preparation containing aspirin. Although the treatment usually simply involves avoidance, desensitisation can be done with success but this is only available in specialist centres.

Desensitisation for this asthma is done using small doses of aspirin given orally, the patient being closely monitored at hospital with repeated breathing tests for some hours after each dose. It is time consuming in the first instance but is worthwhile for some.

Nocturnal asthma

Night-time asthma is often regarded as a particular type of asthma. In fact, waking at night with asthma is an indication of asthma that is poorly controlled overall and applies to any patient with any type of asthma. In most cases appropriate treatment will overcome the problem but some patients are more difficult to control. In these patients, factors such as acid reflux (stomach acid coming back into the chest at night and causing irritation) may be a cause and need treatment. Some drugs, such as theophyllines and the long-acting inhaled bronchodilators, are often helpful in controlling symptoms of nocturnal asthma.

KEY POINTS

✓ A history of allergy may lead to the need for confirmatory tests to identify the allergen

✓ Desensitisation in asthma patients can be dangerous and should only be done in hospital

✓ Patients with brittle asthma should be managed by chest specialists with an interest in the severer forms of asthma

✓ Asthmatic individuals who are sensitive to aspirin should avoid all aspirin-containing drugs. Ask your GP or pharmacist if you are in doubt

✓ Night-time asthma suggests that asthma is poorly controlled

Occupational asthma

Asthma that develops as a result of exposure to a substance or substances at work is regarded as occupational asthma. The exposure may act as an inducer of asthma, where the substance sensitises the patient, who reacts every time he or she is subsequently exposed. Alternatively, the substance may act as an inciter, inducing attacks in patients who already have asthma, which did not necessarily arise originally as a result of the exposure.

Causes of occupational asthma

There are over 200 known causes of occupational asthma, many of them obscure, but some of them occurring in very familiar types of work. They include isocyanates (the hardener in paints used by car body paint sprayers), flour (baker's asthma) and epoxy resins.

A list of the more common causes of occupational asthma is shown on the following page, along with the jobs with which these forms are usually associated.

How common is occupational asthma?

Occupational asthma may affect roughly one in 330 of the working population, or around five per cent of asthmatics at work. These figures are very approximate and are undoubtedly an underestimate of the true amount. Because patients, employers and doctors are often unaware of the possibility that occupational factors could be important, many cases go undiagnosed, which, in some individuals, may be a problem as continued exposure to certain substances can lead to irreversible changes in the airways.

How is occupational asthma diagnosed?

The first clue comes from the patient's history. If your symptoms get better at the weekend or when you are away from work for longer periods, such as holidays, this suggests that something at work may be affecting your asthma. Not all who give such a history do have occupational asthma and, equally, some who don't give such a history do end up with a diagnosis of occupational

Common causes of occupational asthma

Substance	Occupation
Isocyanates	Paint, varnish and some plastic workers
Colophony	Solderers
Animal urine	Laboratory workers, animal breeders
Epoxy resins	Occupations involved with adhesives/varnishes
Flour	Bakery/catering trades
Platinum salts	Refining
Chromium	Tanning, electroplating
Enzymes	Detergent production, drug/food technology
Hardwood dusts	Millers, joiners, carpenters
Nickel	Electroplating
Dyes	Dye manufacture
Antibiotics	Drug manufacturing
Grain mites	Farmers

asthma. However, such a history should result in referral to a chest specialist for further investigations.

After you have been referred to the hospital or chest clinic, the specialist will ask you to record your peak flows regularly, maybe as frequently as every two hours, both when at work and away from work to look for recognisable patterns of change in the peak flow readings that would support the diagnosis.

CASE HISTORY

Brian is 32 years old and has worked in the car industry for 10 years since he had a spell in the Army, where he had begun to learn his trade. For the first four years he had done various jobs around the factory, but he was switched to the paint shop at the age of 26. Although he used to smoke 10 to 15 cigarettes a day, his only problem up to that time had been the occasional bout of winter bronchitis. During the winter of 1990, he had what he thought to be another attack of bronchitis with cough and wheeze, but on this occasion the symptoms persisted and began to wake him at night. He went to his GP who prescribed him another course of antibiotics and told him he really must stop smoking. This had no effect and his wheezing now began to be obvious on even modest

exertion. The GP felt he might have asthma and treated him to some effect shortly before Brian went off on holiday at Easter 1991.

While away, Brian began to feel very much better and even stopped using his inhalers, but as soon as he went back to work his asthma returned with a vengeance. Suspecting that his improvement away from work might imply an occupational aspect to his asthma, his GP referred him to the local chest clinic where serial peak flow readings showed the typical pattern of work-related asthma. Luckily, the firm for which Brian worked was a large concern and they provided him with a very effective protective hood. Since then his asthma has been much easier to control and he has been able to continue work in a job in which he has become skilled and well paid.

Confirming the diagnosis

Occasionally, where there still may be doubt about an occupational origin for your asthma, you may be 'challenged' in the laboratory to the suspected substance under carefully supervised conditions. If you worsen when exposed to the suspect agent but not when exposed – on another day – to another substance not thought to be involved, this will usually clinch the diagnosis. This is a time-consuming process, as you may have to have a week off work, with repeated series of breathing tests being performed after differing exposures in a specially constructed laboratory. There are relatively few of these centres in the UK.

What happens to the patient with occupational asthma?

Some are forced to leave their job, often because their asthma is too difficult to control while they continue to be exposed. In many cases the factory management are either unable or unwilling to improve factory conditions. Some patients are repositioned within the company in a different job where exposure to the offending substance does not occur. Many, however, continue to work and to be exposed, which may be acceptable in some cases if their asthma can be controlled by medication. For those who are forced to leave their employment or are sacked because of poor work attendance, compensation is available for most people through the Industrial Injuries Disablement system. Ask at your Social Security Office for form B1 100(OA) and a reply envelope, and fill in the form. More information can be found in leaflet NI 237, which can be obtained from the same place. If you have any further queries, the staff at the Benefits Agency will be able to help you.

Sometimes, claims for compensation have to go through the courts, which invariably takes time, but may be the only way a skilled worker who has lost a well-paid job can be adequately compensated.

KEY POINTS

✓ Asthma symptoms that improve at the weekend or during holidays suggest an occupational cause

✓ The clue usually comes from the history, but the diagnosis may need to be confirmed in the laboratory

✓ Compensation for those who have to leave their employment is available for most people through the Industrial Injuries Disablement system

Alternative treatments

There is considerable interest in the role of alternative or complementary therapies for the treatment of asthma. This is due to worries about the side-effects of conventional medical treatment and a belief that 'natural substances' are better for asthma than drugs.

Unfortunately, whereas virtually all the available standard treatments for asthma have been proven in properly controlled trials of efficacy, only rarely have complementary approaches been so assessed, which is why many doctors pour scorn on such forms of treatment. Yet complementary practitioners often quote anecdotal stories of benefit and maintain that consis-tent successes over many years show that their treatment works. This has resulted in a polarisation of belief between those who feel that conventional medicine is the only suitable treatment and those who regard conventional treatment as verging on the poisonous! I believe that the truth lies between these two extremes although, predictably, I place more belief in standard medical treatment for asthma.

Nevertheless, the patient needs to be regarded as a whole and not just as 'a case of asthma': his or her beliefs need to be considered and discussed and, very often, where beliefs are strongly held on both sides, compromises can be made, deals can be struck. It must always be remembered that the aim is to control asthma or at least reduce it to an acceptable level in the patient's eyes.

Acupuncture

There is no doubt that acupuncture has found more acceptance in medical circles than have other forms of complementary therapy, particularly with regard to pain relief. It is also one of the few alternative approaches that has been properly tested in clinical tests in asthma. Minor benefits have been shown in the milder forms of asthma, but acupuncture has not been shown to be of help in patients with more severe asthma.

Homoeopathy

There are homoeopathic remedies for chronic asthma which are claimed to work. However, the more strict homoeopaths tell me that their treatment will only be effective if the patient stops taking his or her conventional medication – something I could never condone.

Hypnosis

Some patients claim great benefits from hypnosis, particularly in the way they are able to cope with acute attacks or worsening asthma. For those who believe in this approach, it may be of help, but as with homoeopathy, it would be very helpful to see properly conducted trials of its effect, which, to date, are lacking.

Herbalism

Herbalists often target their therapy on symptoms rather than the condition itself. So if cough is a predominant symptom of asthma, specific attempts to reduce sputum production will be made, often with suggestions for dietary control.

Speleotherapy

I have put this in more to make a point than to recommend it as a possible approach for the British asthmatic patient.

Speleotherapy involves patients spending time, often quite long periods, underground in caves! It appears to work, almost certainly because the patient has been removed from exposure to the house dust mite and other allergens. It is similar to the finding that spending time at altitude helps the bad asthmatic – again due to reduced exposure to the house dust mite.

So environmental control, when it involves removing the patient from exposure to allergens, can help. The problem is finding such an environment to live in!

Summary

Conventional therapy must remain the mainstay for the treatment of asthma in the long term but in some patients who wish to explore alternative therapies, the benefits may be significant.

One important point that must be made is that patients should not simply stop their conventional treatment and switch to an alternative therapy. This has resulted in marked deterioration in some patients who have tried such a wholesale change.

Whether any benefit from complementary measures is due to an effect of belief on such a suggestible condition as asthma or to a direct effect on asthmatic airways is open to debate; perhaps that debate should be encouraged at a more scientific level than it has been in the past.

KEY POINTS

✓ Alternative therapies do appear to help some patients. Whether this is due to their belief in the effectiveness of the alternative approach or to a direct effect on asthmatic airways has not been established

✓ With the exception of acupuncture, the benefits of complementary approaches have rarely been tested in properly controlled trials

The future

So what does the future hold for the patient with asthma? First, there is no doubt that asthma is not going to disappear. It is very common and is likely to remain at current levels for the forseeable future. Deaths from asthma will still occur.

This all sounds very pessimistic but there are a number of lights in the darkness which potentially hold out hope for patients with asthma.

Prevention

It is likely that we will become better at controlling exposure to allergens, and this will be especially important in the first five years of life, when sensitisation to the house dust mite in particular occurs. Such control will require considerable effort on the part of the individual patient or parent!

What we, as doctors, have to do is come up with a package of control measures that are practical and not cripplingly expensive. So far, we have fallen short of this ideal.

Other environmental control measures are needed, notably a reduction in parental smoking, which is so important in the development of asthma in children. There is no easy way to achieve this.

However, there are distinct signs that pollution control measures for towns are being considered which, in time, will improve air quality and could lead to a reduction in the number of asthma attacks.

Treatment

Producing a drug for any new condition is a long and costly business, requiring stringent animal and human studies that have to satisfy the Committee on Safety of Medicines that the drug is both useful and safe. Only then will they provide a product licence for the drug.

So what new drugs are getting through this series of hoops that might be of help to asthmatic patients in the near future?

New tablets

Interestingly, some of the new drugs on the horizon are in tablet form. After all, inhalers can be a nuisance – they are often tricky to use well and only rarely get used as regularly as doctors would like to believe.

The new drugs soon to appear on the market are largely preventive in type, are often in tablet form to be taken twice or even just once a day and have a low frequency of re-corded side-effects. It is probable that they will be more effective in patients with milder asthma but we will have to wait and see what the results of trials show. Certainly, they have the potential to make asthma control easier, more acceptable and with few side-effects.

It is likely that, in the longer term, very specific treatments, per-haps aimed at particular groups of asthmatic patients, will become available.

Whether these will be in inhaled or tablet form will depend on many things, not the least of which will be what patients prefer!

Vaccines

The possibility of being immunised 'against allergy' as opposed to being desensitised against specific allergens is being investigated. This sounds attractive but trials are awaited to see

if this therapy is safe, practical and effective.

Immunisation against those viruses

Again, trials will be necessary to prove that they can reduce attacks and do so safely.

Gene therapy

Although great strides are being made in unravelling the genetics of asthma, particularly with respect to allergy, the possibility of gene therapy is a long way off.

Potentially, this could have almost the greatest effect on asthma but there are many hurdles, both ethical and scientific, to be overcome before that time.

Conclusion

I am optimistic about the future for the asthmatic patient. The development of drugs with fewer side-effects or, better still, improved ways of preventing asthma or asthma attacks will come and will reduce the discomfort you and other asthma sufferers endure today.

that most frequently cause asthma attacks – largely the common cold viruses (rhinoviruses) – may become a distinct possibility in the future once an appropriate vaccine, or vaccines, become available.

KEY POINTS

✓ New tablets are being tested that have the potential to make asthma control easier, more acceptable and with fewer side-effects

✓ Asthma will not be 'eradicated'; however, attempts to prevent rather than treat asthma should be effective in asthma control in the UK

How to use your inhaler

How to use a metered dose inhaler

1 Remove the cap and shake the inhaler.

2 Breathe out gently.

3 Put the mouthpiece in the mouth, and at the start of inspiration, which should be slow and deep, press the canister down and continue to inhale deeply.

4 Hold the breath for 10 seconds or as long as possible.

5 Wait for 30 seconds before taking another inhalation.

A metered dose inhaler

If in doubt always seek professional advice

Reproduced by kind permission of the National Asthma & Respiratory Training Centre.

How to use the Autohaler device

1 Remove the protective mouthpiece and shake the inhaler.

2 Hold the inhaler upright and push the lever right up.

3 Breathe out gently. Keep the inhaler upright and put the mouthpiece in the mouth and close the lips around it (the air holes must not be blocked by the hand).

4 Breath in steadily through the mouth. DON'T stop breathing when the inhaler 'clicks' and continue taking a really deep breath.

5 Hold the breath for about 10 seconds.

6 Note: the lever must be pushed up (on) before each dose, and pushed down again (off) afterwards otherwise it will not operate.

Autohaler

If in doubt always seek professional advice

Reproduced by kind permission of the National Asthma & Respiratory Training Centre.

How to use the Easi-Breathe

1 Shake the inhaler.

2 Hold the inhaler upright. Open the cap.

3 Breathe out gently. Keep the inhaler upright, put the mouthpiece in the mouth and close the lips and teeth around it (the air holes must not be blocked by the hand).

4 Breathe in steadily through the mouthpiece. DON'T stop breathing when the inhaler 'puffs' and continue taking a really deep breath.

5 Hold the breath for about 10 seconds.

6 After use, hold the inhaler upright and immediately close the cap.

7 For a second dose, wait a few seconds before repeating steps 1–6.

Easi-Breathe

If in doubt always seek professional advice

Reproduced by kind permission of the National Asthma & Respiratory Training Centre.

How to use the Accuhaler

1 Hold the outer casing of the Accuhaler in one hand while pushing the thumbgrip away until a click is heard.

2 Hold Accuhaler with mouthpiece towards you; slide lever away until it clicks. This makes the dose available for inhalation and moves the dose counter on.

3 Holding Accuhaler level, breathe out gently away from the device; put mouthpiece in mouth and suck in steadily and deeply.

4 Remove Accuhaler from mouth and hold breath for about 10 seconds.

5 To close, slide thumbgrip back towards you as far as it will go until it clicks.

6 For a second dose repeat steps 1–5.

Accuhaler

If in doubt always seek professional advice

Reproduced by kind permission of the National Asthma & Respiratory Training Centre.

How to use the Turbohaler

1 Unscrew and lift off the white cover. Hold the Turbohaler upright and twist the grip forwards and backwards as far as it will go. You should hear a click.

2 Breathe out gently, put the mouthpiece between the lips and breathe in as deeply as possible. Even when a full dose is taken there may be no taste.

3 Remove the Turbohaler from the mouth and hold the breath for about 10 seconds. Replace the white cover.

Turbohaler

If in doubt always seek professional advice

Reproduced by kind permission of the National Asthma & Respiratory Training Centre.

How to use the Diskhaler

To load

1 Remove mouthpiece cover. Then remove white tray by pulling it out gently and then squeezing white ridges either side until it slides out.

2 Put foil disc – numbers uppermost – on wheel and slide tray back.

3 Holding the corners of the tray, slide tray in and out to rotate disc until number 8 shows in the window

To use

1 Keep the Diskhaler level, lift rear of lid as far up as it will go, to pierce top and bottom of blister. Close the lid.

2 Holding the Diskhaler level, breathe out gently, put mouthpiece in mouth and breathe in as deeply as possible (do not cover the small air holes either side of the mouthpiece).

3 Remove the Diskhaler from the mouth and hold the breath for about 10 seconds. Slide tray in and out ready for the next dose.

Diskhaler

If in doubt always seek professional advice

Reproduced by kind permission of the National Asthma & Respiratory Training Centre.

How to use the Rotahaler

1 Hold the Rotahaler vertically, and put capsule **coloured end uppermost** into the 'square' hole. Make sure the top of the Rotacap is level with the top of the hole (if there is already a Rotacap in the device this will be pushed into the shell).

2 Hold the Rotahaler horizontally; twist barrel sharply forwards and backwards. This splits the capsule into two.

Rotahaler

3 Breathe out gently,
Keep Rotahaler level and
put the mouthpiece between
the lips and teeth and breathe in
the powder quickly and deeply.

4 Remove Rotahaler from the mouth
and hold the breath for about
10 seconds.

If in doubt always seek professional advice

Reproduced by kind permission of the National Asthma & Respiratory Training Centre.

How to use the Spinhaler

1 Hold the Spinhaler upright. with the mouthpiece downwards, and unscrew the body.

2 Put **coloured** end of Spincap **into cup** of propeller, making sure it spins freely.

3 Screw the two parts together, and move the grey sleeve up and down twice; this will pierce the capsule.

4 Breathe out gently, tilt the head back, put the Spinhaler into the mouth so the lips touch the flange, breathe in quickly and deeply.

5 Remove the Spinhaler from the mouth. Hold breath for about 10 seconds and then breathe out slowly.

6 If any powder is left in the Spincap repeat steps 4 & 5 until it is empty.

Spinhaler

If in doubt always seek professional advice

Reproduced by kind permission of the National Asthma & Respiratory Training Centre.

How to use the Aerohaler

To load

1 Open the mouthpiece by lifting it up.

2 Lift the magazine up slightly and turn it round in a clockwise direction until the mark $\overset{6}{\blacktriangledown}$ lines up with Δ on the base. Push the magazine down again.

3 Load the capsules (either way up) into the magazine. Push down the mouthpiece until it clicks.

To use

1 Hold the inhaler upright, Push the white button on the side of the inhaler until it clicks and then release it immediately (this pierces the capsule).

2 Breathe out fully. Put the mouthpiece in the mouth and breathe in as deeply as possible.

3 Remove Aerohaler from the mouth and hold breath for about 10 seconds. Breathe out slowly through the nose.

4 Turn the magazine until the next lowest number appears above the mark Δ on the base. The next dose is then ready.

Aerohaler

If in doubt always seek professional advice

Reproduced by kind permission of the National Asthma & Respiratory Training Centre.

How to use a large volume spacer device

Method for patients who can use the device without help

1 Remove the cap, shake the inhaler and insert into the device.

2 Place the mouthpiece in the mouth.

3 Press the canister once to release a dose of the drug.

4 Take a deep slow breath in.

5 Hold breath for about 10 seconds, then breathe out through the mouthpiece.

6 Breathe in again, but do not press the canister.

7 Remove the device from the mouth.

8 Wait about 30 seconds before a second dose is taken.

Volumatic

If in doubt always seek professional advice

Reproduced by kind permission of the National Asthma & Respiratory Training Centre.

Questions & answers

● **Will the asthma go?**
This is the question most commonly asked by parents about their child with asthma. Most children of primary school age appear to lose their asthma, often in their teens, so a condition that is more common in boys becomes slightly more common in adult women. This is not to say that the asthma has disappeared for ever, as a proportion of patients suffer a relapse in later life – in women this is often around the time of the menopause. Sometimes, the symptoms of the newly returned asthma are different from those experienced as a child – wheezing will often be more common in childhood, and breathlessness and chest tightness more common in adulthood.

Most people who develop asthma in adult life will retain it to a greater or lesser degree for the rest of their lives. It is not clear what proportion who develop asthma in adulthood lose it, but a reasonable estimate would be around only 20 per cent.

● **Will the asthma or treatment damage the lungs?**
Patients believe that 'the lungs' are different from 'the tubes' whereas the tubes are a part of the lungs. The worry about long-term damage is, however, a real one. Undertreated, asthma can lead to irreversible narrowing of the airways because the inflammation is not being controlled. Similarly, patients who smoke and don't use their preventive inhaler regularly may develop quite severe irreversible damage to their lungs.

The treatment for asthma does not damage the lungs although steroid tablets can cause many other side-effects, as discussed on pages 42–4.

Taken overall, the risks of damage to the individual are greater with untreated asthma than when the asthma is controlled.

● **Will the treatment wear off?**
The drug treatment for asthma does not wear off. If you find that your relief inhaler is becoming less effec-

tive, this is far more likely to be due to worsening asthma than the drug itself having no effect. The drug may be finding it more difficult to work at that dose or, because the airways are narrower as the asthma worsens, less will be getting to the lower airways. If you find that your treatment is becoming less effective, it is essential that you go to your doctor for reassessment. It is not true that taking a certain dose of an inhaler will lead to you needing a progressively higher dose as the years go by.

● **Is asthma catching?**
No it is not. Asthma is not an infectious disease and cannot be caught from another person.

● **Are nebulisers dangerous?**
A nebuliser is a powerful way of delivering drugs to the lungs and is therefore used only in the patient with more severe asthma. Nevertheless, there are some patients using nebuliser therapy for whom other forms of treatment haven't been fully explored. When used only for acute attacks, nebulisers can save lives and admission to hospital. The danger

comes when too much reliance is placed on the 'all-powerful' nebuliser and instead of seeking medical help, the patient self-administers repeated nebulised doses. This can lead to a very severe, even life-threatening, episode, which could have been avoided had the patient gone to casualty or contacted their GP.

Once a patient is established on regular nebulised therapy, clearly his or her asthma is bad. Many will never be able to stop the treatment, unless a new treatment, which may be perfect for them, comes along. Occasionally, changes in circumstances, such as a move to a different part of the country, or removal from an occupational cause, can result in marked improvement in their asthma and they may then not need to use their nebuliser.

Again, as with other forms of inhaled therapy, using nebulised therapy under good supervision will not mean that you will need higher and higher doses as the years go by. If that appears to be happening it is more likely to be due to the asthma itself worsening than an effect of the nebulised drug.

Useful addresses

National Asthma Campaign (NAC)

This is the only charity solely dedicated to asthma. It raises funds for research and is the biggest contributor to asthma research in the UK. It has an active network of local groups run by asthmatics for asthmatics who provide a variety of services to their local population apart from raising remarkable amounts of money for research. It was formed by the amalgamation of the Asthma Society and the Asthma Research Council.

NAC
Providence House
Providence Place
Islington
London N1 0NT.
Tel: 0171 226 2260
Asthma Helpline: 0345 010203

The British Allergy Foundation (BAF)

This organisation was founded in June 1991 by a group of leading medical specialists determined to improve the awareness, prevention and treatment of allergy. The British Allergy Foundation encompasses all types of allergy and aims to offer information and support to sufferers as well as raising funds for allergy-related research. Work is mainly funded by voluntary income and a small government grant towards the cost of the Allergy Helpline.

British Allergy Foundation
30 Bellegrove Road
Welling
Kent
DA16 3BY
Tel: 0181 303 8525
Allergy Helpline: 0181 303 8583

The National Asthma and Respiratory Training Centre

This centre was established as a result of the need for increasing the ability of general practices to manage asthma without needing to refer to hospital. The centre trains nurses to manage asthma in the general practice and chest clinic setting by a combination of a distance learning package and a residential course. Their results have been phenomenal in improving the quality of asthma care delivered to patients today.

National Asthma and
Respiratory Training Centre
Atheneaum
10 Church Street
Warwick CV34 4AB
Tel: 01926 493313
Fax: 01926 493224

The British Lung Foundation
This charity was established in 1985 to raise funds for research into all forms of lung disease. They also have a series of self-help groups around the country, 'The Breathe Easy Club',

largely run by patients.

British Lung Foundation
78 Hatton Garden
London EC1N 8JR
Tel: 0171 831 5831

The Anaphylaxis Campaign
Information on peanut/food anaphy-laxis (that is to say, immediate allergic reaction) – please send an s.a.e.

The Anaphylaxis Campaign
PO Box 149
Fleet
Hants GU13 9XU
Tel: 01252 318723

Index